Culinary Healing for Pancreatitis

Wholesome Recipes and Nutrient-Packed Strategies for Wellness

Zara Lackey

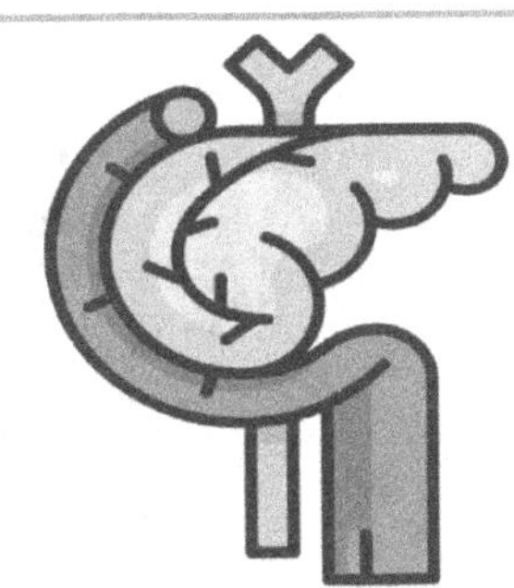

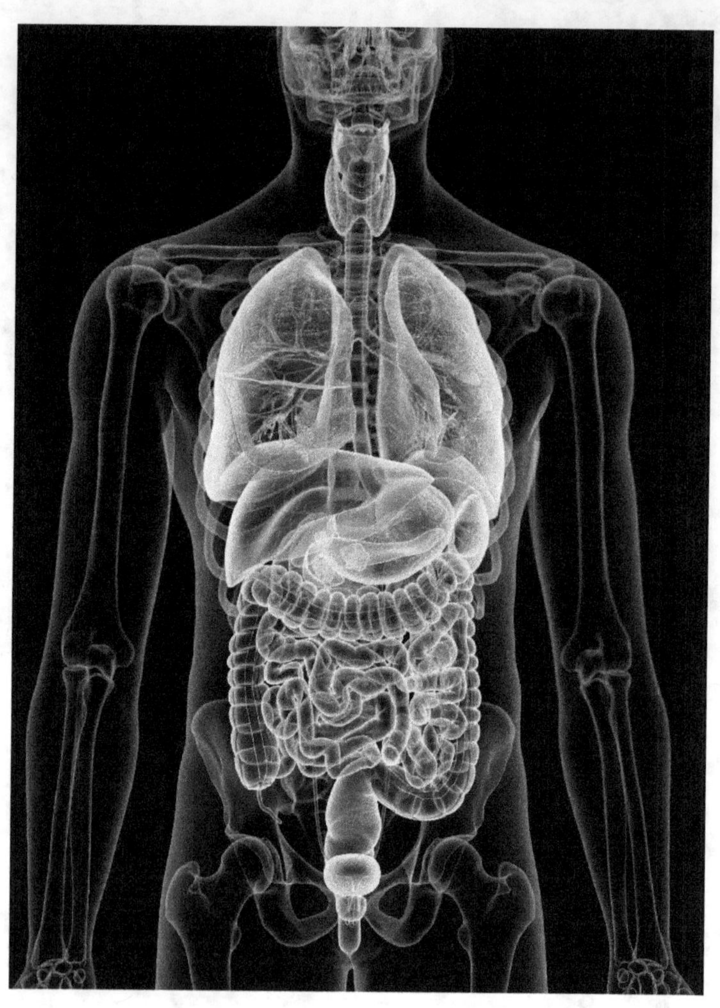

Disclaimer

Dedication

To those navigating the path of pancreatitis with resilience and determination,
This cookbook is dedicated to each individual facing the challenges of pancreatitis with unwavering strength. Your journey is marked by courage, and this collection of recipes is crafted to be a companion on your road to wellness. May these flavors bring comfort, nourishment, and joy to your table. Your tenacity inspires us, and this book is a tribute to your perseverance.

With heartfelt wishes for health and healing,

[Zara]

Table of contents

Introduction

In the quiet moments of life, where the aroma of a home-cooked meal lingers, and the gentle sizzle of a pan speaks of warmth, there exists a profound connection between nourishment and well-being. Our journey into the world of healing recipes for pancreatitis begins not with medical jargon or dietary prescriptions but with a story, a story that echoes the shared struggles and triumphs of individuals facing the challenge of managing pancreatitis.

Natasha, a resilient soul whose path to healing intertwined with the comforting embrace of wholesome cooking. Her journey was not just about mastering recipes; it was a profound exploration of how food, thoughtfully chosen and lovingly prepared, could become a source of healing. Sarah's kitchen transformed into a sanctuary where each ingredient held the promise of wellness, and every meal became a gesture of self-care.

Through this cookbook, we invite you to discover not only the science behind pancreatitis-friendly diets but also the heartfelt narratives of those, like Natasha, who found solace and strength in the act of preparing and savoring meals tailored to their well-being. It is a celebration of resilience, a testament to the healing power of food, and a guide that transcends the kitchen, reaching into the hearts of those seeking a brighter, healthier tomorrow.

In the tapestry of life, health, and well-being, the thread of our choices often weaves the most intricate patterns. This cookbook, "Culinary Healing for Pancreatitis: Wholesome Recipes and Nutrient-Packed Strategies for Wellness," embarks on a journey that delicately intertwines the elements of compassion, culinary artistry, and the resilience of the human spirit.

A. Overview of Pancreatitis

Pancreatitis, a condition that touches the lives of many, is often a silent struggle. The pancreas, a small but mighty organ, plays a crucial role in our digestive system.

Yet, when affliction strikes, it demands attention and care. In the pages that follow, we delve into the nuances of this condition, shedding light on its impact and the courage it takes to navigate its challenges.

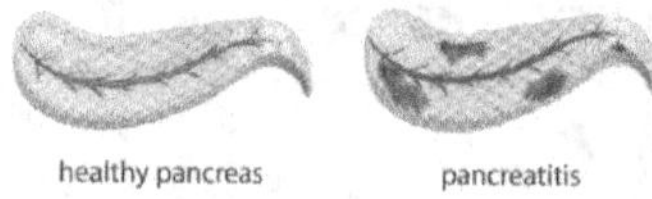

B. Importance of Diet in Managing Pancreatitis

Amidst the complexities of managing pancreatitis, the significance of diet emerges as a beacon of hope. Every morsel becomes an opportunity for healing, and each meal becomes a gesture of self-love. Understanding the profound connection between diet and well-being becomes a cornerstone in the journey toward recovery.

C. How This Cookbook Can Help

This cookbook is more than a collection of recipes, it's a guide crafted with care and empathy.

It seeks to empower individuals facing pancreatitis by providing not just nourishing recipes but also a roadmap to culinary well-being. From the intricacies of dietary guidelines to the comforting allure of kitchen essentials, each chapter is a step towards not just managing pancreatitis but embracing a lifestyle that fosters holistic health.

As we embark on this culinary odyssey, let each chapter be a testament to the transformative power of food, the joy of cooking, and the resilience that blooms in the heart of those on the path to wellness. Welcome to a world where healing is an art, and every bite is a step towards rejuvenation.

Join us on this culinary journey, a journey that goes beyond recipes, creating a tapestry of flavors, stories, and well-being.

Chapter One

Understanding Pancreatitis Diets

In the intricate tapestry of managing pancreatitis, knowledge becomes a potent tool. This chapter delves into the core aspects of understanding pancreatitis diets, offering a comprehensive guide to navigating dietary guidelines, nutritional requirements, and the nuanced art of meal planning and preparation.

A. Dietary Guidelines for Pancreatitis

1. Low-Fat Embrace

- Pancreatitis often calls for a reduction in fat intake. Opt for lean protein sources such as skinless poultry, fish, and legumes.

- Limit saturated and trans fats, found in fried foods and processed snacks, as they can trigger pancreatic inflammation.

2. Balanced Nutrition

- Prioritize a well-balanced diet with an emphasis on fruits, vegetables, whole grains, and lean proteins.

- Explore anti-inflammatory foods like berries, spinach, and nuts, known for their potential to alleviate pancreatitis symptoms.

3. Mindful Eating

- Practice mindful eating to enhance digestion. Chew food thoroughly and savor each bite, reducing the workload on the pancreas during the digestive process.

B. Nutritional Requirements and Restrictions

1. Protein Prowess

- Adequate protein intake is crucial for healing. Incorporate sources like Greek yogurt, eggs, and tofu into your diet.

- Consider consulting a healthcare professional or nutritionist to determine your personalized protein needs.

2. Vitamin and Mineral Focus

- Pay attention to vitamin and mineral intake, especially A, D, E, and K, as these are fat-soluble and may be affected by reduced fat absorption.

- Consider supplements or foods rich in these vitamins, such as fortified cereals and leafy greens.

3. Hydration Essentials

- Stay well-hydrated to support digestion. Water, herbal teas, and clear broths are excellent choices.

- Monitor caffeine and alcohol intake, as they can contribute to dehydration.

C. Tips for Meal Planning and Preparation

1. Small and Frequent

- Opt for smaller, more frequent meals to ease the digestive burden on the pancreas.

- Example: Plan five to six small meals/snacks throughout the day, incorporating nutrient-dense foods.

2. Cooking Techniques

- Embrace low-fat cooking methods such as baking, grilling, steaming, and sautéing.
- Instead of frying, try oven-baked chicken seasoned with herbs.

3. Label Literacy

- Scrutinize food labels for hidden fats, sugars, and additives.
- Choose plain yogurt over flavored varieties to avoid added sugars.

4. Meal Timing Considerations

- Allow time between eating and bedtime to aid digestion. Aim for at least two hours.
- Schedule dinner earlier in the evening, and consider a light snack if needed before bedtime.

Navigating the intricacies of pancreatitis diets requires a blend of knowledge, creativity, and mindful choices. By understanding dietary guidelines, nutritional needs, and adopting smart meal planning, you pave the way for a nourishing and supportive culinary journey.

Chapter Two

Kitchen Essentials for Pancreatitis-Friendly Cooking

Embarking on a journey of culinary healing for pancreatitis extends beyond the recipes themselves, it begins in the heart of your kitchen. This chapter unravels the essential elements of a pancreatitis-friendly culinary haven, from low-fat cooking techniques to well-stocked pantries and utensils that make meal preparation a seamless joy.

A. Low-Fat Cooking Techniques

1. Baking Brilliance

- Utilize baking as a wholesome alternative to frying. Bake lean proteins like chicken or fish for a delightful, low-fat option.

- Prepare a succulent piece of cod seasoned with herbs, baked to perfection.

2. Grilling Goodness

- Elevate flavors without excess fat by grilling vegetables, lean meats, or even fruit for a unique twist.

- Grill colorful bell peppers alongside skinless turkey burgers for a flavorful and low-fat meal.

3. Steaming Simplicity

- Preserve nutrients and keep things light by incorporating steaming. Vegetables, rice, and even fish can be steamed with ease.

- Steam a medley of broccoli, carrots, and cauliflower as a vibrant side dish.

4. Sautéing Sensibility

- Opt for sautéing with heart-healthy oils like olive oil in moderation. This technique adds depth without excessive fat.

- Sauté diced onions and garlic in olive oil before adding vegetables for a flavorful base.

B. Essential Pantry Items

1. Whole Grains Galore

- Stock up on whole grains like quinoa, brown rice, and oats for a fiber-rich foundation to your meals.
- Create a nourishing bowl with quinoa as a base, topped with grilled chicken and colorful vegetables.

2. Lean Protein Cornerstones

- Maintain a variety of lean proteins such as canned tuna, beans, and skinless poultry for versatile and protein-packed options.
- Prepare a quick salad with canned chickpeas, cherry tomatoes, and a drizzle of balsamic vinaigrette.

3. Herb and Spice Collection

- Enhance flavors without excess salt or fat by cultivating a diverse herb and spice collection.
- Elevate a simple roasted sweet potato with a sprinkle of cinnamon and a dash of nutmeg.

4. Healthy Fat Sources

- Include sources of healthy fats like avocados, nuts, and seeds to add richness without overwhelming the pancreas.
- Blend avocado into a creamy dressing for a nutrient-packed salad.

C. Cooking Utensils for Easy Meal Preparation

1. Sharp and Trusty Knives
- Invest in sharp knives for precise and effortless chopping, reducing the time spent in meal preparation.
- Example: Slice through vegetables with ease, ensuring consistent sizes for even cooking.

2. Non-Stick Cookware
- Choose non-stick cookware to minimize the need for excessive cooking oils.
- Example: Prepare an egg-white omelet without worrying about sticking to the pan.

3. Food Processor Magic
- Harness the efficiency of a food processor for chopping, blending, and pureeing ingredients with minimal effort.
- Example: Create a smooth hummus by blending chickpeas, tahini, and lemon juice in a food processor.

4. Steamer Basket Convenience

- Integrate a steamer basket for quick and efficient steaming of vegetables and grains.
- Example: Steam broccoli florets to perfection for a nutrient-rich side dish.

As you curate your kitchen for pancreatitis-friendly cooking, let these essentials become the foundation of a culinary sanctuary where healing flavors and practical tools converge. With low-fat techniques, a well-stocked pantry, and efficient utensils, you set the stage for a nourishing and enjoyable cooking experience.

Chapter Three

Breakfast Delights

Mornings, with their quiet promise of a new day, offer an opportunity to kickstart your well-being with wholesome and pancreatitis-friendly breakfasts. This chapter unfolds delightful options, from the heartiness of oatmeal with fresh fruit to the savory delight of scrambled egg whites with vegetables and the refreshing simplicity of a low-fat yogurt parfait.

A. Oatmeal with Fresh Fruit

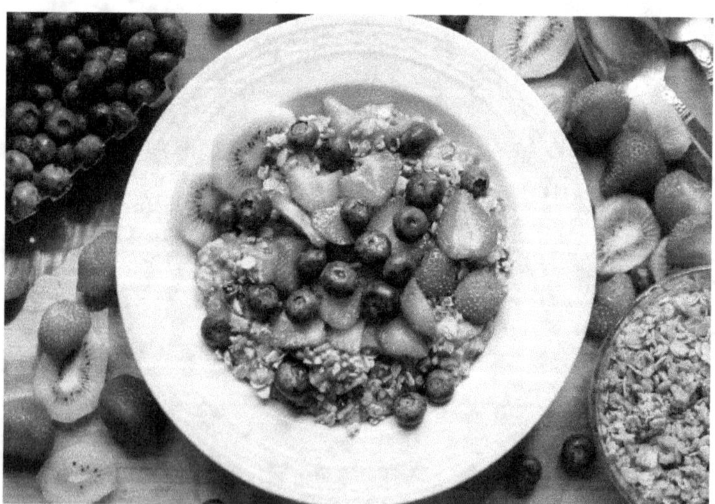

Ingredients

- 1 cup rolled oats
- 2 cups water or low-fat milk
- Pinch of salt
- Fresh fruit of your choice (e.g., berries, sliced banana)
- 1 tablespoon honey or maple syrup (optional)
- Nuts or seeds for topping (optional)

Prep Time: 5 minutes
Cook Time: 10 minutes
Servings: 2

Preparation

1. In a saucepan, bring water or milk to a gentle boil.
2. Stir in the rolled oats and a pinch of salt.
3. Reduce heat to a simmer, stirring occasionally until the oats are creamy and fully cooked.
4. Serve in bowls, top with fresh fruit, and drizzle with honey or maple syrup if desired.
5. Garnish with nuts or seeds for added texture.

Nutritional Value (per serving)

- Calories: 250
- Protein: 8g
- Fiber: 5g
- Healthy fats: 3g
- Carbohydrates: 45g

B. Scrambled Egg Whites with Vegetables

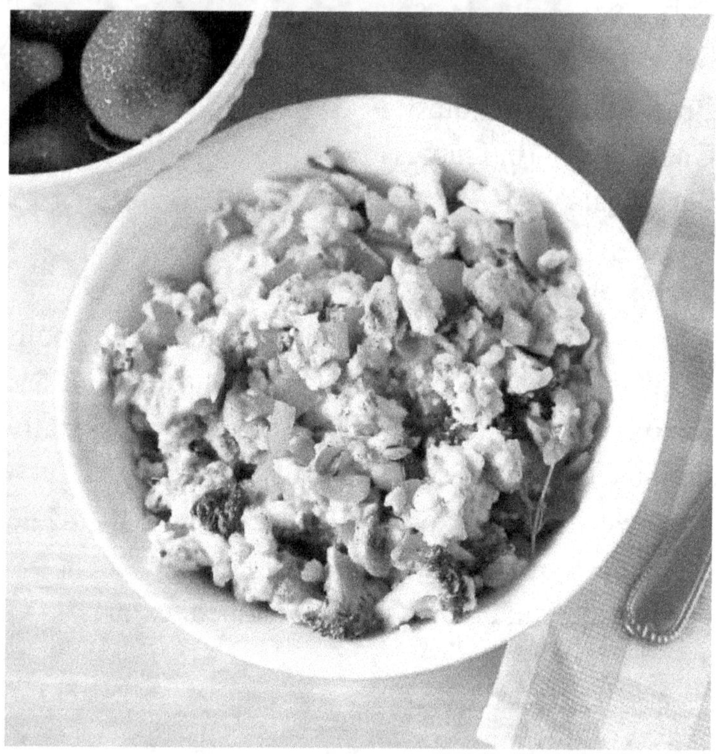

Ingredients

- 4 egg whites
- 1/2 cup diced bell peppers (assorted colors)
- 1/4 cup diced onions
- 1/4 cup spinach, chopped
- Salt and pepper to taste
- Cooking spray or a teaspoon of olive oil

Prep Time: 10 minutes
Cook Time: 5 minutes
Servings: 2

Preparation

1. Heat a non-stick skillet over medium heat and coat with cooking spray or a small amount of olive oil.
2. Sauté diced bell peppers and onions until softened.
3. Add chopped spinach and continue cooking until wilted.
4. Whisk egg whites in a bowl, season with salt and pepper, and pour over the vegetables.
5. Gently scramble until the eggs are fully cooked.
6. Serve hot.

Nutritional Value (per serving)

- Calories: 120
- Protein: 18g
- Fiber: 3g
- Healthy fats: 1g
- Carbohydrates: 9g

C. Low-Fat Yogurt Parfait

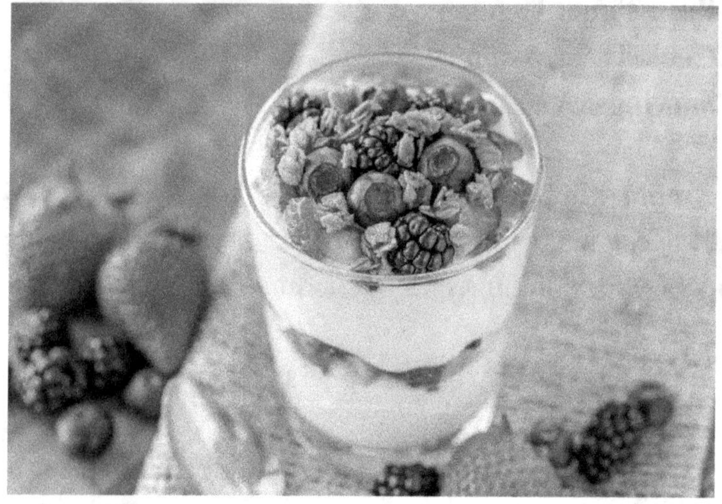

Ingredients

- 1 cup low-fat Greek yogurt
- 1/2 cup granola (choose a low-fat, low-sugar option)
- Fresh berries (e.g., strawberries, blueberries)
- 1 tablespoon honey

Prep Time: 5 minutes

Servings: 1

Preparation
1. In a glass or bowl, layer half of the Greek yogurt.
2. Add a layer of granola, followed by fresh berries.
3. Repeat the layers.
4. Drizzle with honey for a touch of sweetness.

Nutritional Value (per serving)
- Calories: 300
- Protein: 20g
- Fiber: 5g
- Healthy fats: 5g
- Carbohydrates: 40g

These breakfast delights not only tantalize your taste buds but also provide essential nutrients to kickstart your day with energy and nourishment. Experiment with toppings and flavors to tailor them to your preferences while adhering to pancreatitis-friendly guidelines.

Chapter Four

Lunchtime Favorites

As the sun climbs high, lunchtime beckons with an array of flavorful options that not only satisfy your palate but also align with pancreatitis-friendly principles. This chapter explores the crisp freshness of a Grilled Chicken Salad, the wholesome goodness of a Quinoa and Vegetable Bowl, and the delightful portability of a Turkey and Avocado Wrap.

A. Grilled Chicken Salad

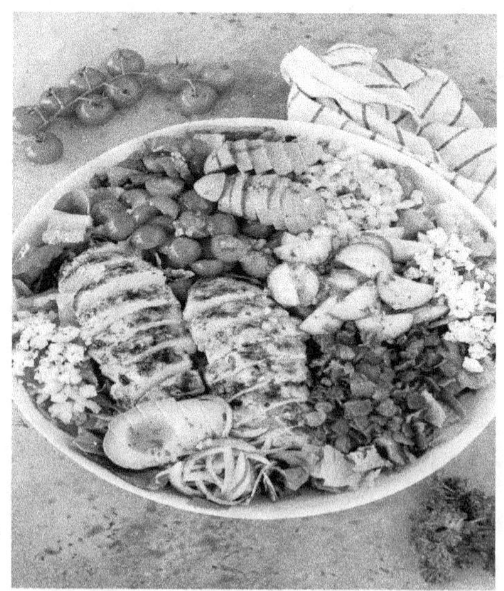

Ingredients

- 2 boneless, skinless chicken breasts
- Mixed salad greens (e.g., spinach, arugula, romaine)
- Cherry tomatoes, halved
- Cucumber, sliced
- Red onion, thinly sliced
- Balsamic vinaigrette dressing
- Olive oil, for grilling
- Salt and pepper to taste

Prep Time: 15 minutes
Cook Time: 15 minutes
Servings: 2

Preparation

1. Season chicken breasts with salt and pepper.
2. Grill the chicken over medium heat until fully cooked, approximately 7-8 minutes per side.
3. Let the chicken rest for a few minutes before slicing it into strips.
4. In a large bowl, toss the mixed salad greens, cherry tomatoes, cucumber, and red onion.
5. Arrange the grilled chicken strips on top.
6. Drizzle with balsamic vinaigrette dressing and toss gently.

7. Serve immediately.

Nutritional Value (per serving)
- Calories: 300
- Protein: 30g
- Fiber: 5g
- Healthy fats: 10g
- Carbohydrates: 20g

B. Quinoa and Vegetable Bowl

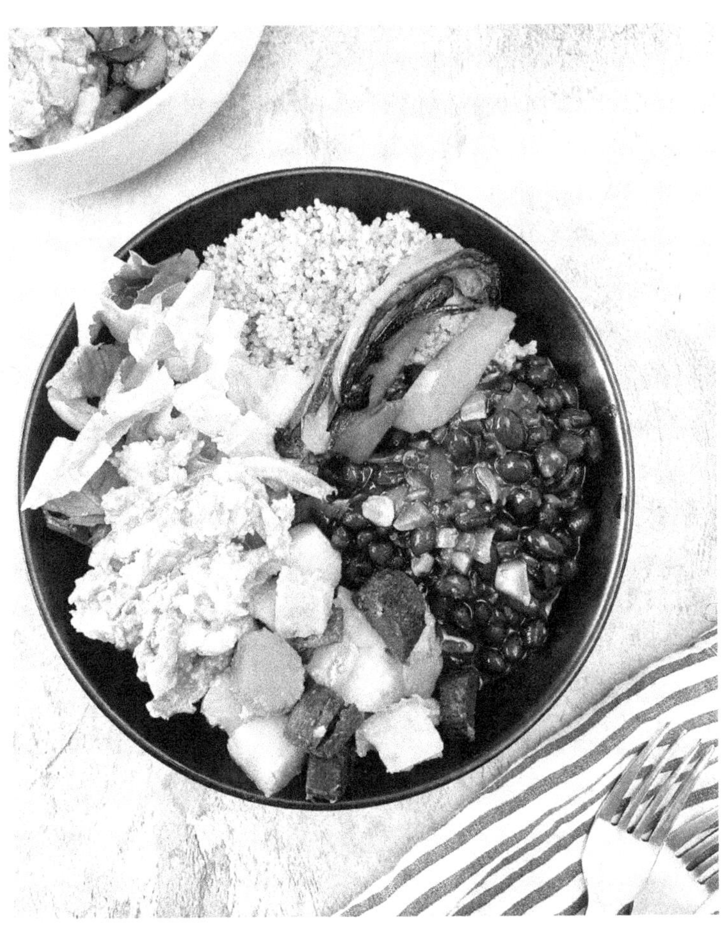

Ingredients

- 1 cup cooked quinoa
- Mixed vegetables (e.g., bell peppers, zucchini, cherry tomatoes)
- Chickpeas, drained and rinsed
- Feta cheese, crumbled
- Olive oil
- Lemon juice
- Fresh herbs (e.g., parsley, mint)
- Salt and pepper to taste

Prep Time: 20 minutes
Cook Time: 15 minutes
Servings: 2

Preparation

1. Cook quinoa according to package instructions.
2. In a pan, sauté mixed vegetables until tender.
3. In a bowl, combine cooked quinoa, sautéed vegetables, chickpeas, and crumbled feta cheese.
4. Drizzle with olive oil and lemon juice.
5. Toss in fresh herbs and season with salt and pepper.
6. Mix well and serve.

Nutritional Value (per serving)

- Calories: 400

- Protein: 15g
- Fiber: 10g
- Healthy fats: 15g
- Carbohydrates: 50g

C. Turkey and Avocado Wrap

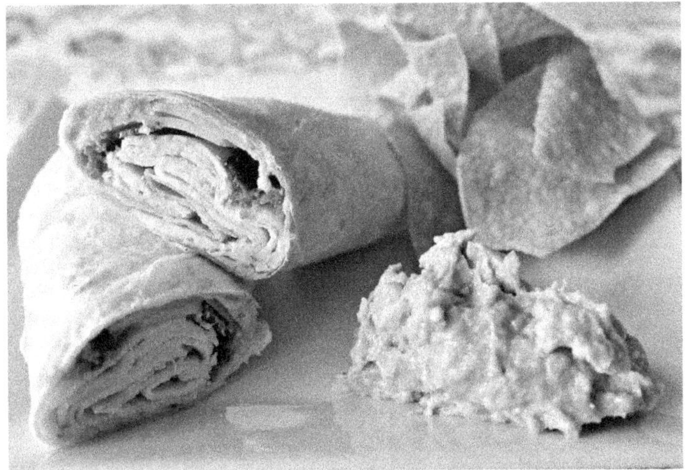

Ingredients

- 8 oz. lean turkey slices
- Whole-grain or spinach tortillas
- Avocado, sliced
- Mixed greens
- Cherry tomatoes, halved
- Greek yogurt or a light dressing
- Salt and pepper to taste

Prep Time: 10 minutes
Servings: 2

Preparation
1. Lay out tortillas and layer with turkey slices.
2. Add sliced avocado, mixed greens, and cherry tomatoes.
3. Drizzle with Greek yogurt or a light dressing.
4. Season with salt and pepper.
5. Wrap tightly and slice in half.
6. Serve immediately.

Nutritional Value (per serving)
- Calories: 350
- Protein: 25g
- Fiber: 8g
- Healthy fats: 15g
- Carbohydrates: 30g

These lunchtime favorites offer a symphony of flavors and textures while adhering to pancreatitis-friendly guidelines. Whether you crave the crunch of a salad, the heartiness of quinoa, or the convenience of a wrap, these options make lunch a satisfying and nutritious experience.

Chapter Five

Dinner Creations

As the day draws to a close, these dinner creations offer a delightful array of flavors and textures, all while adhering to the principles of pancreatitis-friendly cooking. From the succulence of Baked Salmon with Lemon and Dill to the vibrant Stir-Fried Tofu and Vegetables and the wholesome Roasted Sweet Potato and Black Bean Bowl, these recipes promise both nourishment and satisfaction.

A. Baked Salmon with Lemon and Dill

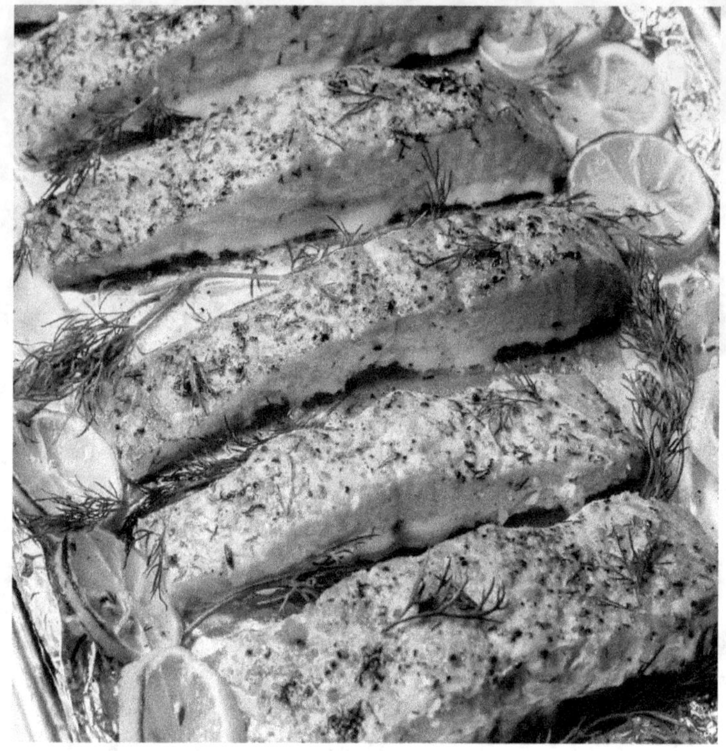

Ingredients

- 2 salmon fillets
- Fresh dill, chopped
- Lemon slices
- Olive oil
- Garlic powder
- Salt and pepper to taste

Prep Time: 10 minutes

Cook Time: 15 minutes
Servings: 2

Preparation
1. Preheat the oven to 400°F (200°C).
2. Place salmon fillets on a baking sheet lined with parchment paper.
3. Drizzle with olive oil and season with garlic powder, salt, and pepper.
4. Top with fresh dill and lemon slices.
5. Bake in the preheated oven for 12-15 minutes or until the salmon is cooked through.
6. Serve hot.

Nutritional Value (per serving)
- Calories: 350
- Protein: 30g
- Healthy fats: 20g
- Omega-3 fatty acids: 1.5g
- Carbohydrates: 2g

B. Stir-Fried Tofu and Vegetables

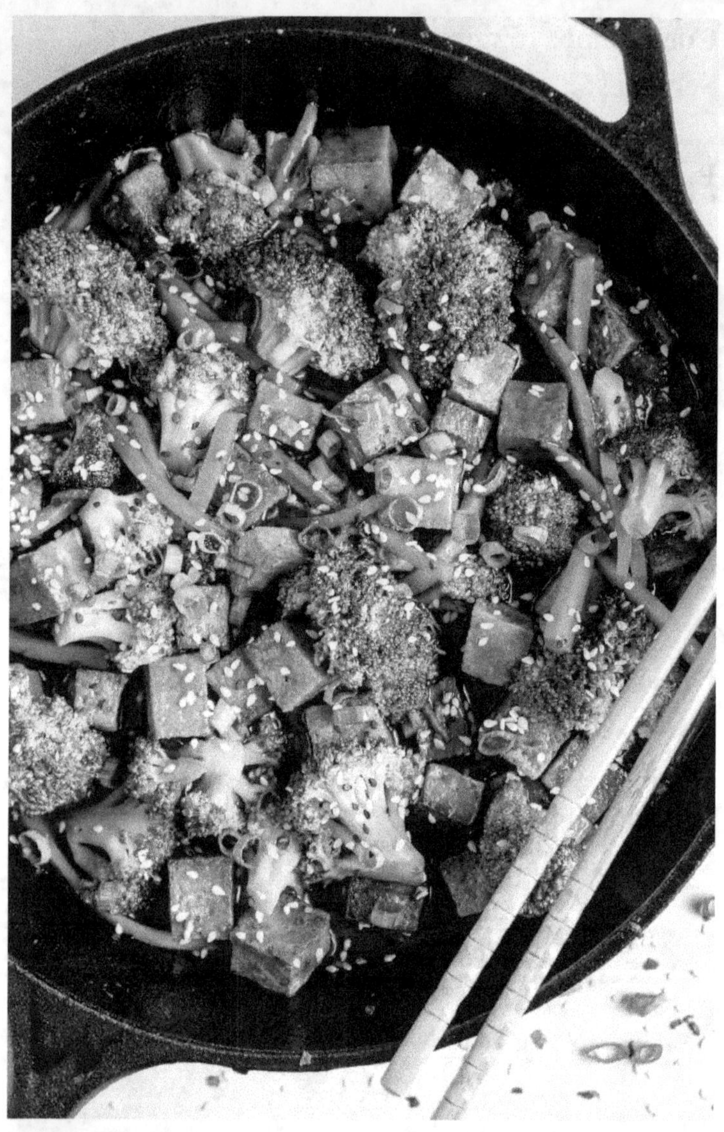

Ingredients

- 14 oz. extra-firm tofu, pressed and cubed

- Mixed vegetables (e.g., broccoli, bell peppers, snap peas)
- Soy sauce
- Sesame oil
- Ginger, minced
- Garlic, minced
- Green onions, chopped
- Sesame seeds (optional)

Prep Time: 20 minutes
Cook Time: 15 minutes
Servings: 2

Preparation

1. In a wok or skillet, heat sesame oil over medium-high heat.
2. Add cubed tofu and stir-fry until golden brown on all sides.
3. Remove tofu from the wok and set aside.
4. In the same wok, stir-fry mixed vegetables, ginger, and garlic until crisp-tender.
5. Add the cooked tofu back to the wok and drizzle with soy sauce.
6. Garnish with chopped green onions and sesame seeds.
7. Serve over rice or quinoa.

Nutritional Value (per serving)
- Calories: 300
- Protein: 20g
- Healthy fats: 15g
- Carbohydrates: 25g
- Fiber: 8g

C. Roasted Sweet Potato and Black Bean Bowl

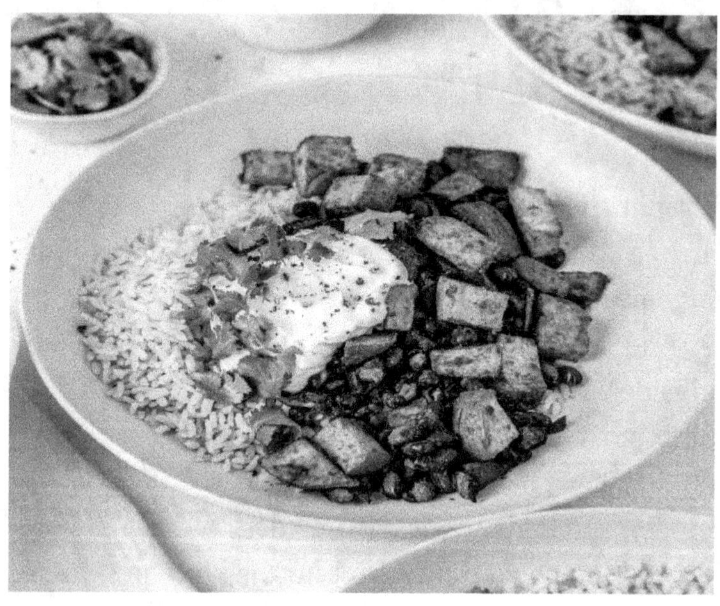

Ingredients
- 2 medium sweet potatoes, peeled and cubed

- 1 can (15 oz.) black beans, drained and rinsed
- Olive oil
- Smoked paprika
- Cumin
- Chili powder
- Salt and pepper to taste
- Avocado, sliced (optional)
- Fresh cilantro, chopped (optional)

Prep Time: 15 minutes
Cook Time: 30 minutes
Servings: 2

Preparation
1. Preheat the oven to 400°F (200°C).
2. In a bowl, toss sweet potato cubes with olive oil, smoked paprika, cumin, chili powder, salt, and pepper.
3. Spread the seasoned sweet potatoes on a baking sheet and roast for 25-30 minutes or until tender.
4. In a separate bowl, mix black beans with a dash of cumin and chili powder.
5. Assemble bowls with roasted sweet potatoes and seasoned black beans.

6. Garnish with sliced avocado and chopped fresh cilantro if desired.

Nutritional Value (per serving)
- Calories: 380
- Protein: 12g
- Healthy fats: 10g
- Carbohydrates: 65g
- Fiber: 15g

These dinner creations not only showcase diverse culinary techniques but also provide a rich tapestry of nutrients to round off your day in a delicious and wholesome manner. Whether you savor the omega-3 richness of baked salmon, the protein-packed stir-fry, or the comforting warmth of a roasted sweet potato bowl, these recipes bring dinner to life in a nourishing and pancreatitis-friendly way.

Chapter Six

Snacks and Appetizers

Between meals, these snacks and appetizers invite you to indulge in flavors that not only satisfy cravings but also align with the principles of pancreatitis-friendly eating. From the vibrant Fresh Fruit Salsa with Baked Pita Chips to the classic Hummus and Veggie Platter and the energy-boosting Nut and Seed Mix, these recipes promise delightful moments of nibbling.

A. Fresh Fruit Salsa with Baked Pita Chips

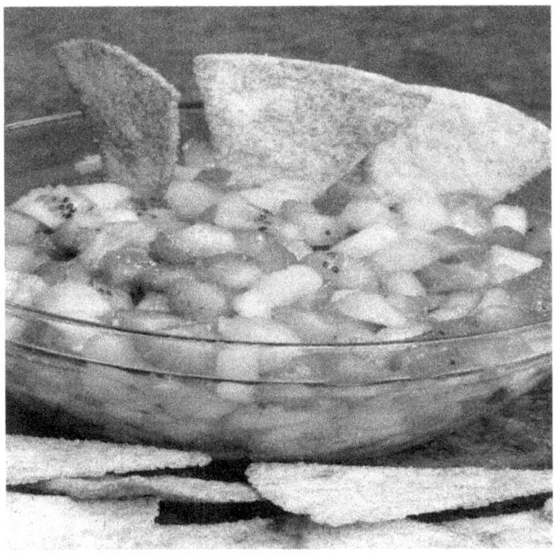

Ingredients

- 2 cups mixed fresh fruits (e.g., strawberries, mango, kiwi), diced
- 1 tablespoon fresh mint, chopped
- 1 tablespoon honey or agave syrup
- Zest and juice of one lime
- Whole-grain pita bread

Prep Time: 15 minutes
Cook Time: 10 minutes
Servings: 4

Preparation

1. Preheat the oven to 350°F (180°C).
2. Cut whole-grain pita bread into triangles.
3. Arrange the triangles on a baking sheet and bake for 8-10 minutes or until crisp.
4. In a bowl, combine diced fresh fruits, chopped mint, honey or agave syrup, lime zest, and lime juice.
5. Mix gently and let it sit for a few minutes.
6. Serve the fruit salsa with the baked pita chips.

Nutritional Value (per serving)

- Calories: 150
- Fiber: 5g
- Vitamins: A, C
- Antioxidants: Flavonoids

B. Hummus and Veggie Platter

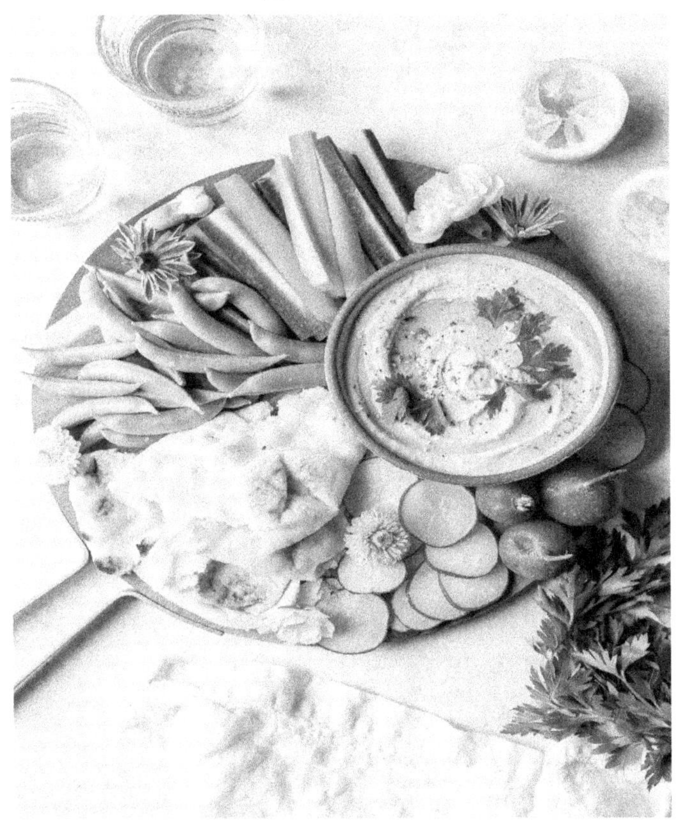

Ingredients
- 1 cup hummus
- Carrot sticks
- Cucumber slices
- Cherry tomatoes, halved
- Bell pepper strips (assorted colors)
- Whole-grain crackers or rice cakes

Prep Time: 10 minutes
Servings: 4

Preparation
1. Arrange hummus in the center of a serving platter.
2. Surround it with carrot sticks, cucumber slices, cherry tomatoes, and bell pepper strips.
3. Add whole-grain crackers or rice cakes for dipping.
4. Serve chilled.

Nutritional Value (per serving)
- Calories: 200
- Protein: 8g
- Fiber: 6g
- Healthy fats: 10g
- Vitamins: A, C

C. Nut and Seed Mix

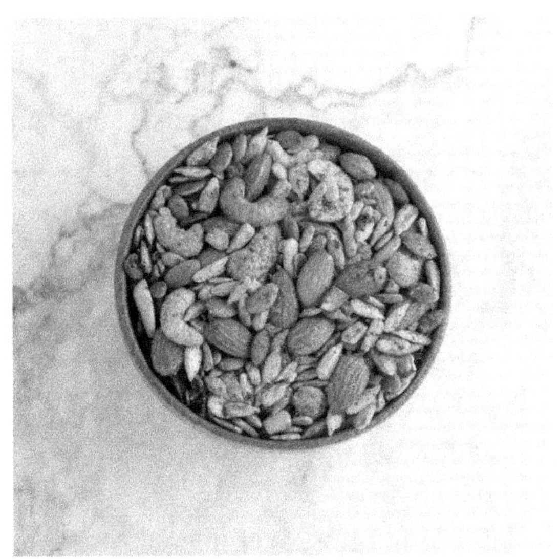

Ingredients

- 1/2 cup almonds
- 1/2 cup walnuts
- 1/4 cup pumpkin seeds
- 1/4 cup sunflower seeds
- 1 tablespoon chia seeds
- 1 tablespoon flaxseeds
- 1 teaspoon olive oil
- Pinch of sea salt

Prep Time: 10 minutes
Cook Time: 0 minutes
Servings: 4

Preparation

1. In a dry skillet over medium heat, lightly toast almonds, walnuts, pumpkin seeds, and sunflower seeds until fragrant (about 3-5 minutes).

2. In a bowl, combine toasted nuts and seeds with chia seeds and flaxseeds.

3. Drizzle with olive oil and sprinkle with a pinch of sea salt.

4. Toss to coat evenly.

5. Allow the mix to cool before serving.

Nutritional Value (per serving)

- Calories: 250
- Protein: 8g
- Fiber: 6g
- Healthy fats: 20g
- Omega-3 fatty acids: 1.5g

These snacks and appetizers transform the mundane into moments of culinary delight. Whether you're savoring the sweetness of Fresh Fruit Salsa, indulging in the classic combination of Hummus and Veggies, or enjoying the crunchy Nut and Seed Mix, these recipes ensure that your snacking experiences are both flavorful and nourishing.

Chapter Seven

Beverages for Pancreatitis

Hydration and refreshment take center stage in this chapter, offering a delightful array of beverages that not only quench your thirst but also align with the principles of pancreatitis-friendly nutrition. From the revitalizing Infused Water Recipes to the soothing Herbal Teas and their benefits, and the nutrient-packed indulgence of Smoothies, these beverages promise a flavorful journey of hydration.

A. Infused Water Recipes

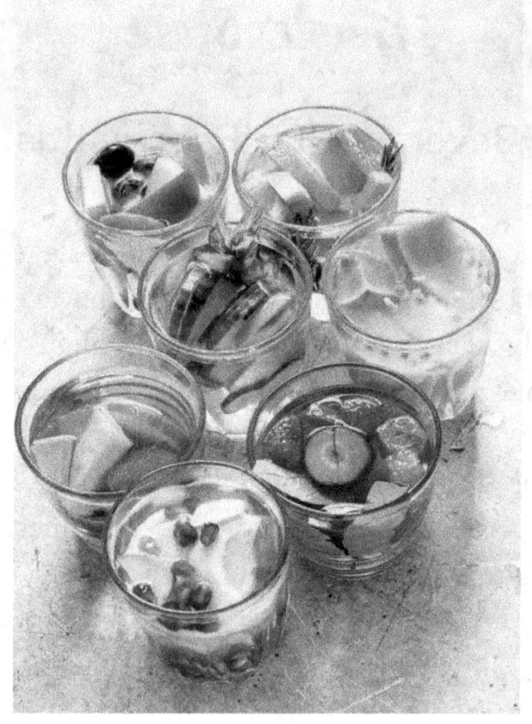

Ingredients

- Option 1: Cucumber and Mint
- 1/2 cucumber, thinly sliced
- Fresh mint leaves
- Option 2: Citrus Burst
- Slices of orange, lemon, and lime
- Fresh basil leaves
- Option 3: Berry Bliss
- Mixed berries (e.g., strawberries, blueberries, raspberries)

- Basil or rosemary sprigs
- Cold water and ice cubes

Prep Time: 5 minutes
Servings: 2

Preparation
1. Choose your infusion ingredients and add them to a pitcher.
2. Fill the pitcher with cold water and add ice cubes.
3. Allow the water to infuse for at least 1-2 hours in the refrigerator.
4. Serve chilled.

B. Herbal Teas and Their Benefits

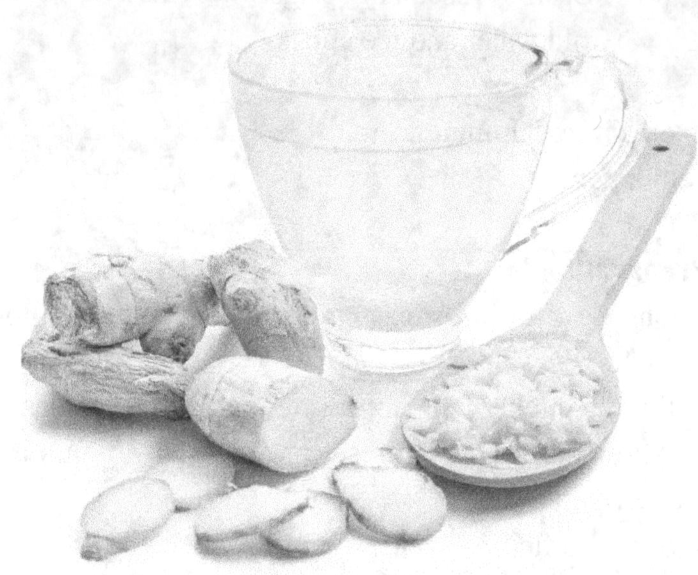

Ingredients

- Chamomile tea bags
- Peppermint tea bags
- Ginger tea bags or fresh ginger slices
- Hot water

Prep Time: 5 minutes
Cook Time: 5 minutes
Servings: 2

Preparation

1. Choose your herbal tea blend.

2. Place tea bags or fresh ginger slices in a teapot or cup.
3. Pour hot water over the tea bags or ginger.
4. Allow the tea to steep for 5 minutes.
5. Remove tea bags or strain out ginger.
6. Serve warm.

Herbal Tea Benefits
- Chamomile: Soothing and anti-inflammatory.
- Peppermint: Aids digestion and provides a refreshing flavor.
- Ginger: Anti-inflammatory and may help with nausea.

C. Smoothies for a Nutrient Boost

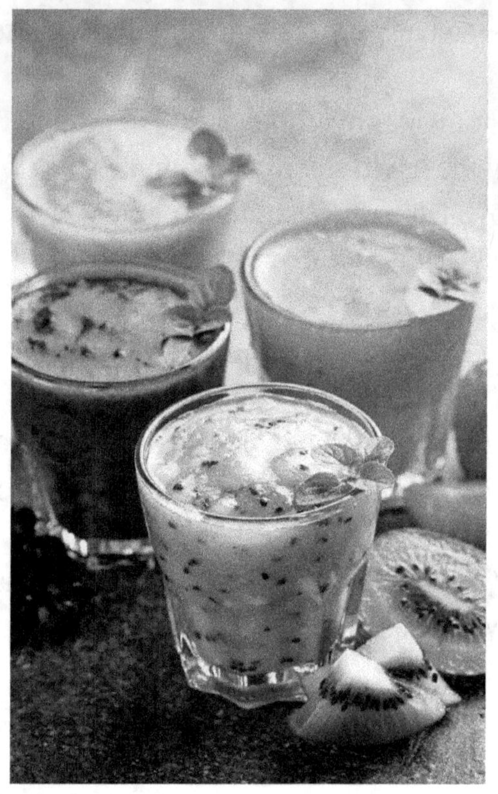

Ingredients

- Option 1: Green Goodness
- Handful of spinach
- 1/2 banana
- 1/2 cup pineapple chunks
- 1/2 cup coconut water
- Option 2: Berry Blast
- Mixed berries (e.g., blueberries, raspberries, strawberries)

- 1/2 cup Greek yogurt
- Almond milk
- Option 3: Tropical Paradise
- Mango chunks
- Pineapple slices
- 1/2 cup coconut milk
- Ice cubes

Prep Time: 10 minutes
Servings: 2

Preparation
1. Choose your smoothie blend and add ingredients to a blender.
2. Blend until smooth and creamy.
3. Add ice cubes for a refreshing chill.
4. Pour into glasses and enjoy immediately.

Nutritional Value (per serving)
- Calories: 150-200
- Protein: 5-10g
- Fiber: 3-5g
- Vitamins and minerals: Varied based on ingredients

These beverages not only elevate your hydration game but also provide an infusion of flavors and health benefits. Whether you're sipping on the refreshing Infused Water, enjoying the calming properties of Herbal Teas, or indulging in the nutrient-packed goodness of Smoothies, these recipes are designed to complement your pancreatitis-friendly lifestyle.

Chapter Eight

Dessert Delights

Indulge your sweet tooth without compromising on pancreatitis-friendly principles with these dessert delights. From the refreshing Banana and Berry Sorbet to the warm comfort of Baked Apple Slices with Cinnamon, and the luscious Yogurt and Berry Parfait, this chapter promises a satisfying conclusion to your meals.

A. Banana and Berry Sorbet

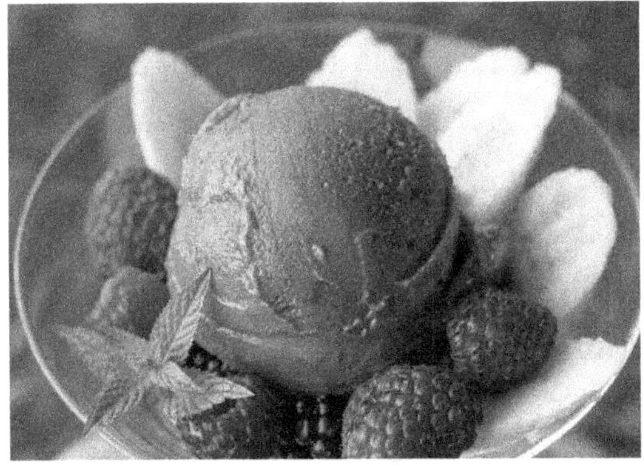

Ingredients

- 2 ripe bananas, peeled and sliced
- 1 cup mixed berries (e.g., strawberries, blueberries, raspberries)
- 1-2 tablespoons honey or agave syrup (optional)
- Juice of half a lemon

Prep Time: 10 minutes
Freeze Time: 4 hours
Servings: 2

Preparation

1. Arrange banana slices and mixed berries on a baking sheet lined with parchment paper.
2. Freeze for at least 4 hours or until solid.
3. Transfer the frozen fruits to a blender or food processor.
4. Add honey or agave syrup and lemon juice.
5. Blend until smooth and creamy.
6. Serve immediately.

Nutritional Value (per serving)

- Calories: 120
- Fiber: 4g
- Vitamins: C, B6

- Antioxidants: Flavonoids

B. Baked Apple Slices with Cinnamon

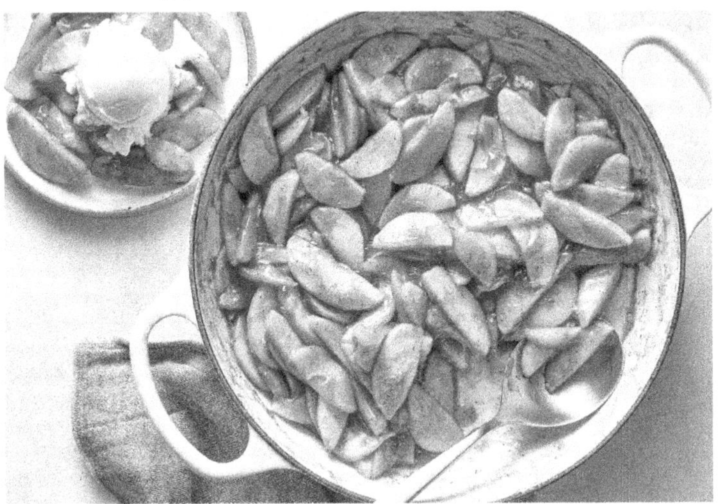

Ingredients

- 2 apples, cored and thinly sliced
- 1 teaspoon ground cinnamon
- 1 tablespoon honey
- Lemon zest (optional)

Prep Time: 10 minutes
Bake Time: 15 minutes
Servings: 2

Preparation

1. Preheat the oven to 375°F (190°C).
2. Toss apple slices with ground cinnamon and honey.
3. Arrange the slices on a baking sheet lined with parchment paper.
4. Bake for 15 minutes or until the apples are tender.
5. Sprinkle with lemon zest if desired.
6. Serve warm.

Nutritional Value (per serving)
- Calories: 80
- Fiber: 4g
- Vitamins: C, K
- Minerals: Potassium

C. *Yogurt and Berry Parfait*

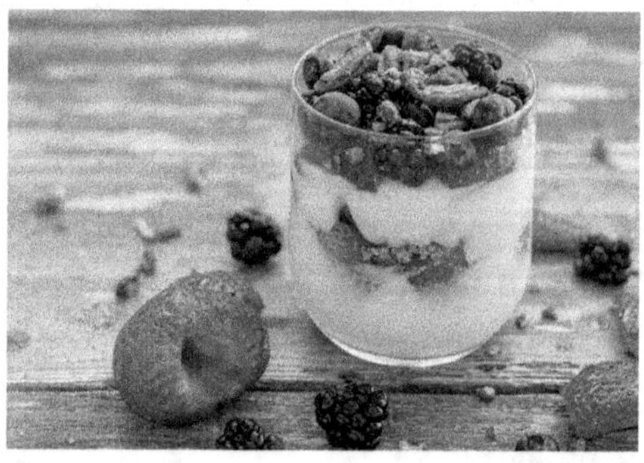

Ingredients

- 1 cup low-fat Greek yogurt
- Mixed berries (e.g., strawberries, blueberries, blackberries)
- Granola (choose a low-fat, low-sugar option)
- 1 tablespoon honey

Prep Time: 10 minutes
Servings: 2

Preparation
1. In a glass or bowl, layer Greek yogurt.
2. Add a layer of mixed berries.
3. Sprinkle granola over the berries.
4. Repeat the layers.
5. Drizzle with honey for sweetness.
6. Serve chilled.

Nutritional Value (per serving)
- Calories: 250
- Protein: 15g
- Fiber: 5g
- Healthy fats: 5g
- Carbohydrates: 40g

These dessert delights offer a symphony of flavors and textures, proving that sweet treats can be both indulgent and pancreatitis-friendly. Whether you're savoring the coolness of Banana and Berry Sorbet, enjoying the warmth of Baked Apple Slices, or delighting in the layers of Yogurt and Berry Parfait, these recipes provide a delightful conclusion to your culinary journey.

Chapter Nine

Meal Plans for Various Dietary Needs

Navigating the landscape of pancreatitis-friendly eating is made easier with tailored meal plans designed to cater to different dietary needs. Whether you're prioritizing a low-fat approach, embracing a vegetarian lifestyle, or navigating the world of gluten-free options, these meal plans provide a roadmap to delicious and pancreatitis-conscious eating.

A. Low-Fat Meal Plan

A low-fat meal plan is crafted to support pancreatitis management by minimizing dietary fat, promoting digestion, and reducing the workload on the pancreas.

Example Day

Breakfast

- Oatmeal with sliced strawberries and a sprinkle of chia seeds.
- Herbal tea or infused water.

Lunch

- Grilled chicken salad with mixed greens, cherry tomatoes, and a light vinaigrette.
- Quinoa and vegetable bowl.

Snack

- Fresh fruit salsa with baked pita chips.

Dinner

- Baked salmon with lemon and dill.
- Steamed broccoli and brown rice.

Dessert

- Banana and berry sorbet.

B. Vegetarian Pancreatitis Meal Plan

A vegetarian meal plan focuses on plant-based sources of protein, incorporating a variety of fruits, vegetables, legumes, and whole grains to promote pancreatitis-friendly nutrition.

Example Day

Breakfast

- Scrambled tofu with spinach and cherry tomatoes.
- Whole-grain toast with avocado.

Lunch

- Quinoa and black bean salad with a lime-cilantro dressing.
- Hummus and veggie platter.

Snack

- Nut and seed mix.

Dinner

- Stir-fried tofu and vegetables with brown rice.
- Roasted sweet potato and black bean bowl.

Dessert

- Yogurt and berry parfait.

C. Gluten-Free Options Meal Plan

A gluten-free meal plan eliminates gluten-containing grains like wheat, barley, and rye, providing alternatives that are kind to the digestive system.

Example Day

Breakfast
- Gluten-free overnight oats with almond milk and sliced peaches.
- Green tea or infused water.

Lunch
- Grilled chicken salad with gluten-free quinoa.

Snack
- Fresh fruit slices with gluten-free nut butter.

Dinner

- Baked salmon with gluten-free breadcrumbs and lemon.
- Steamed asparagus and quinoa.

Dessert

- Baked apple slices with cinnamon.

These meal plans serve as a foundation for crafting diverse and delicious meals while adhering to specific dietary needs. Feel free to customize them based on personal preferences and consult with a healthcare professional or nutritionist for personalized guidance on managing pancreatitis through dietary choices.

Chapter Ten

Tips for Dining Out with Pancreatitis

Dining out with pancreatitis can be a pleasurable experience when armed with knowledge and a proactive approach. This chapter provides detailed insights into making informed menu choices, effectively communicating dietary needs to restaurants, and navigating the challenges of traveling with dietary restrictions.

A. Making Informed Menu Choices

1. Research the Menu
- Before heading to a restaurant, explore their menu online. Look for options that align with pancreatitis-friendly guidelines, such as lean protein, low-fat choices, and well-cooked vegetables.

2. Choose Lean Proteins

- Opt for lean protein sources like grilled chicken, turkey, fish, or tofu. Request preparation methods that involve minimal added fats.

3. Embrace Vegetables and Fruits

- Prioritize dishes featuring a variety of vegetables and fruits. These provide essential nutrients and are often gentle on the digestive system.

4. Avoid Fried and Greasy Foods

- Steer clear of fried and greasy items, as they can be high in fat and may trigger pancreatitis symptoms.

5. Request Modifications

- Don't hesitate to ask for modifications to suit your dietary needs. Restaurants are often willing to accommodate requests, such as using less oil or omitting certain ingredients.

B. Communicating Dietary Needs to Restaurants

1. Be Clear and Specific

- Clearly communicate your dietary restrictions to the server. Specify any ingredients that need to be avoided or modified.

2. Ask About Preparation Methods

- Inquire about how dishes are prepared. Choose options that involve grilling, baking, or steaming rather than frying.

3. Request Sauces and Dressings on the Side

- Ask for sauces, dressings, or condiments on the side. This allows you to control the amount you consume.

4. Inform about Food Allergies

- If you have specific food allergies in addition to pancreatitis, clearly communicate them to the staff to prevent cross-contamination.

5. Express Sensitivity to Spices

- Mention if you are sensitive to spicy foods, as certain spices can be harsh on the digestive system.

C. Traveling with Dietary Restrictions

1. Plan Ahead

- Research restaurants at your travel destination and identify those with pancreatitis-friendly options.

2. Pack Snacks

- Bring pancreatitis-friendly snacks for the journey, ensuring you have readily available and suitable options.

3. Communicate Dietary Needs in Advance

- If possible, inform airlines or hotels about your dietary restrictions in advance. Many establishments are willing to accommodate special requests.

4. Consider Self-Catering Options

- If traveling allows, consider accommodations with kitchen facilities. This enables you to prepare meals that align with your dietary needs.

5. Learn Local Terminology

- Familiarize yourself with local food terms to help navigate menus more effectively in regions where English may not be widely spoken.

By adopting these tips, you can confidently enjoy dining out and traveling while managing pancreatitis. Remember that open communication with restaurant staff is key, and planning ahead can significantly enhance your dining experience and overall well-being.

Chapter Eleven

Conclusion

As you embark on this culinary journey tailored for pancreatitis, this concluding chapter offers a comprehensive overview, encouraging a mindful approach to both cooking and lifestyle choices. Let's recap the principles of pancreatitis-friendly cooking, provide encouragement for a healthier lifestyle, and guide you towards additional resources and support.

A. Recap of Pancreatitis-Friendly Cooking Principles

1. Embrace Lean Proteins
- Prioritize lean protein sources such as poultry, fish, tofu, and legumes. These options provide essential nutrients without overwhelming the pancreas.

2. Choose Low-Fat Cooking Methods

- Opt for cooking methods like grilling, baking, steaming, or sautéing with minimal oil. This reduces the overall fat content in meals.

3. Incorporate Abundant Fruits and Vegetables

- Integrate a colorful array of fruits and vegetables into your diet. They provide vitamins, minerals, and antioxidants while being gentle on the digestive system.

4. Mindful Carbohydrate Choices

- Select whole grains, legumes, and complex carbohydrates. These choices contribute to sustained energy levels without causing spikes in blood sugar.

5. Monitor Portion Sizes

- Pay attention to portion sizes to prevent overeating. Smaller, more frequent meals can be easier on digestion.

B. Encouragement for a Healthier Lifestyle

1. Consistency is Key

- Consistency in following pancreatitis-friendly principles is crucial. Small, sustainable changes over time can lead to significant improvements in overall health.

2. Listen to Your Body

- Pay attention to how your body responds to different foods. Personalized adjustments to your diet based on your unique needs can contribute to better well-being.

3. Stay Hydrated

- Hydration is essential for overall health. Water, herbal teas, and infused waters can contribute to proper hydration without adding unnecessary strain.

4. Incorporate Physical Activity

- Engage in regular, gentle physical activity, such as walking or yoga, to support overall health and well-being.

5. Prioritize Mental Well-Being
- Mental health plays a vital role in overall wellness. Incorporate stress-reducing activities such as meditation, deep breathing, or hobbies you enjoy.

C. Additional Resources and Support

1. Consult with Healthcare Professionals
- Work closely with your healthcare team, including your primary care physician and a registered dietitian. They can provide personalized guidance based on your specific health needs.

2. Seek Support Groups
- Connect with others who are managing pancreatitis through online forums or local support groups. Sharing experiences and tips can provide valuable insights.

3. Explore Educational Materials

- Read reputable books, articles, and websites that focus on pancreatitis management. Staying informed empowers you to make educated decisions about your health.

4. Consider Cooking Classes

- Attend cooking classes or workshops focused on pancreatitis-friendly recipes. Learning new culinary skills can make the journey enjoyable and sustainable.

5. Stay Informed about Research Advances

- Keep abreast of the latest research and medical advances related to pancreatitis. Understanding emerging insights can inform your approach to managing the condition.

As you conclude this cookbook, remember that each meal is an opportunity to nurture your well-being. By embracing pancreatitis-friendly cooking principles, maintaining a holistic and healthier lifestyle, and seeking ongoing support, you empower yourself to thrive on this journey towards wellness. May your culinary adventures be both delicious and nourishing.

Feedback and Reviews:

Your feedback is invaluable. Share your thoughts, suggestions, and reviews online. Your insights not only help improve future editions but also guide others on their journey.

Thank you!

www.ingramcontent.com/pod-product-compliance
Lightning Source LLC
Chambersburg PA
CBHW061012260726
48661CB00005B/2167